EARL STEVENS

Earl Stevens Selections
EARL STEVENS
MANGOSCATO
EARL STEVENS
FUNCTION RED BLEND
CALIFORNIA
EARL STEVENS
MOSCATO
CALIFORNIA
EARL STEVENS

EARL STEVENS
MANGOSCATO

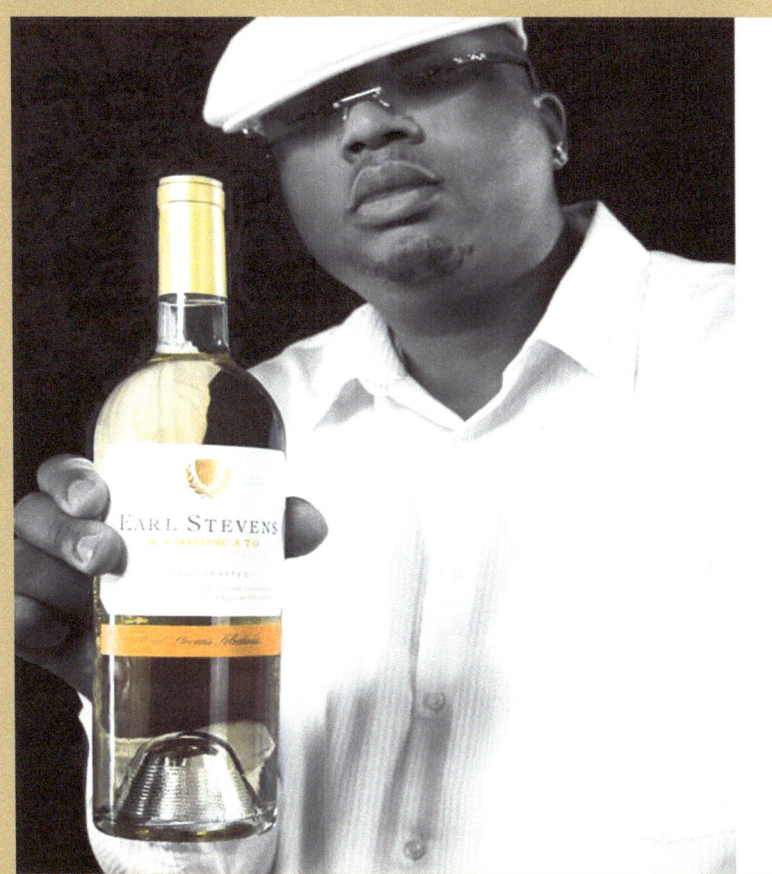

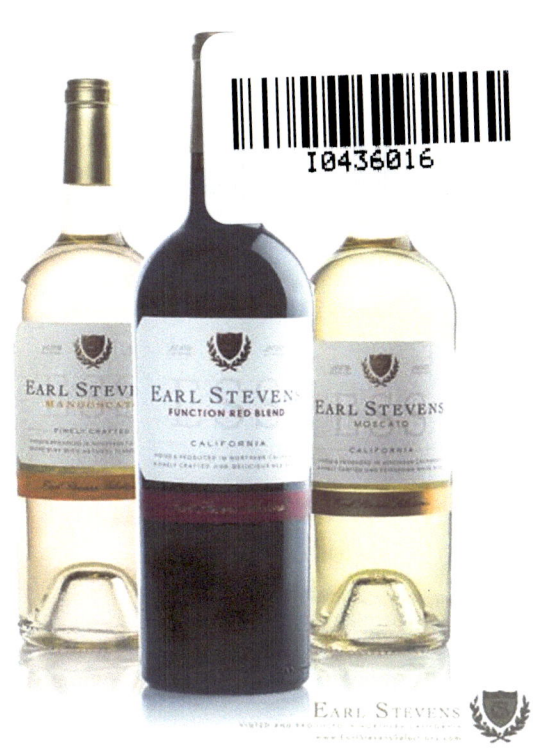

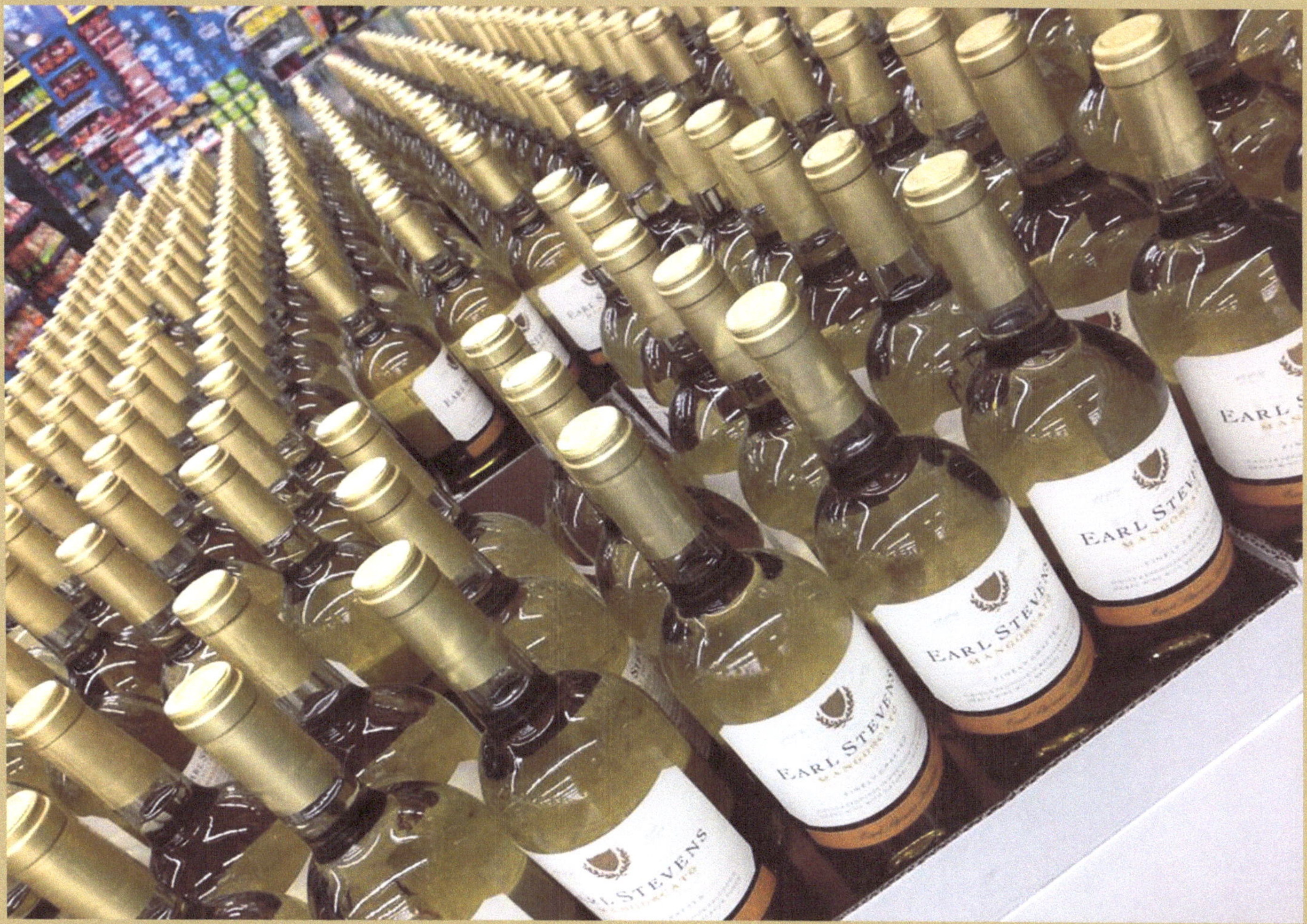

10 Ripped Rappers & Singers

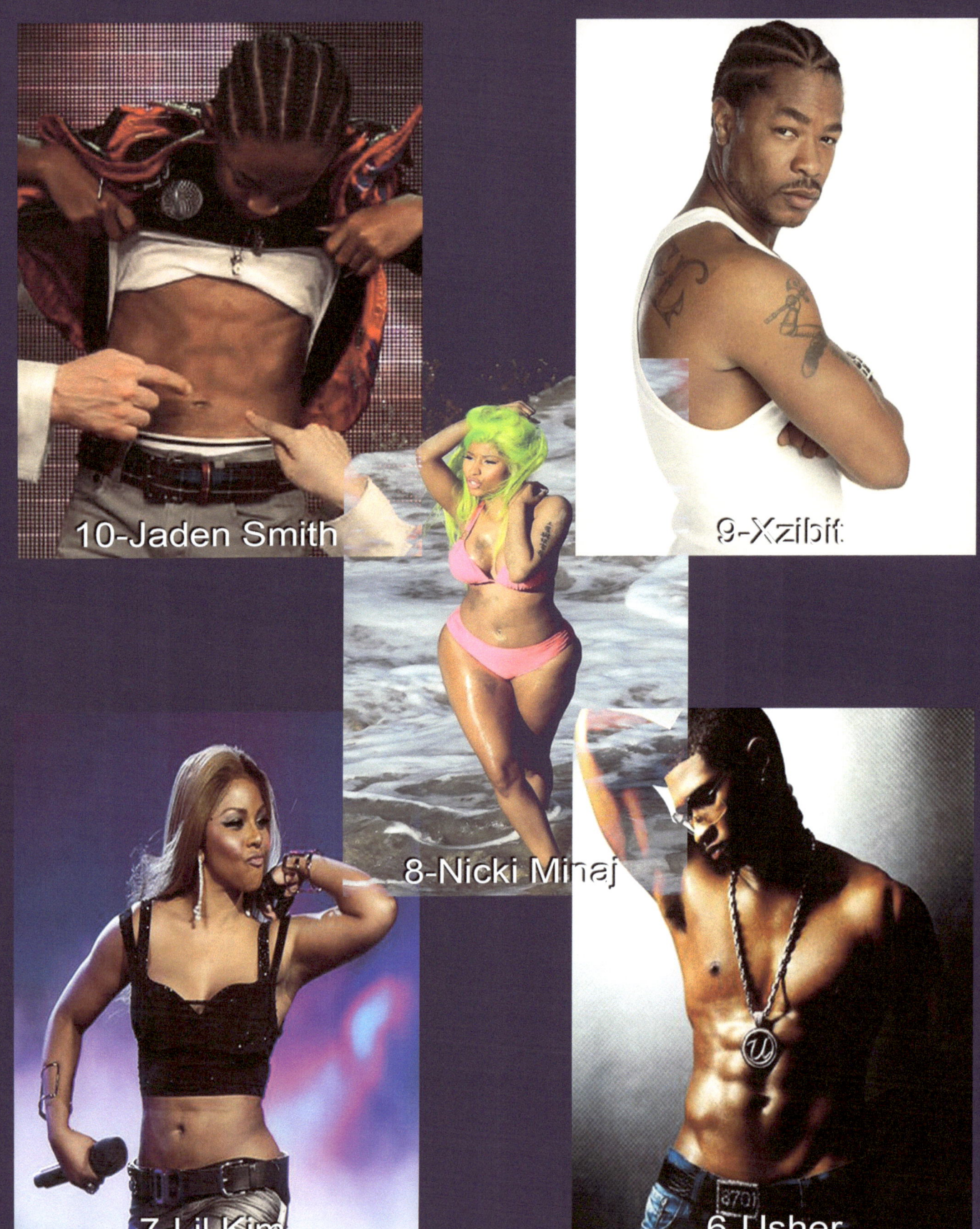

10-Jaden Smith

9-Xzibit

8-Nicki Minaj

7-Lil Kim

6-Usher

10 Ripped Rappers & Singers

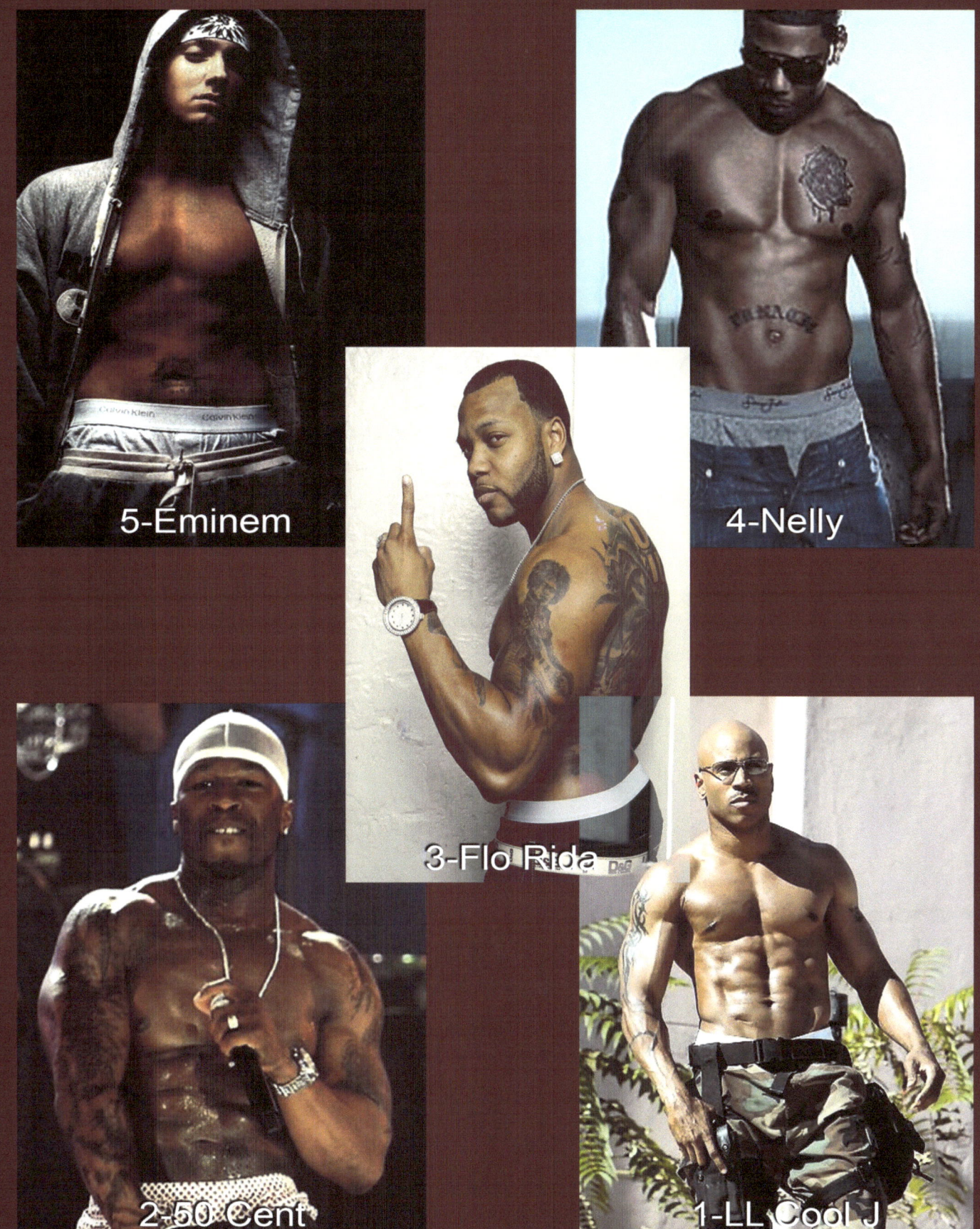

5-Eminem

4-Nelly

3-Flo Rida

2-50 Cent

1-LL Cool J

70-Year-Old Looks 30, Reveals Fountain of Youth

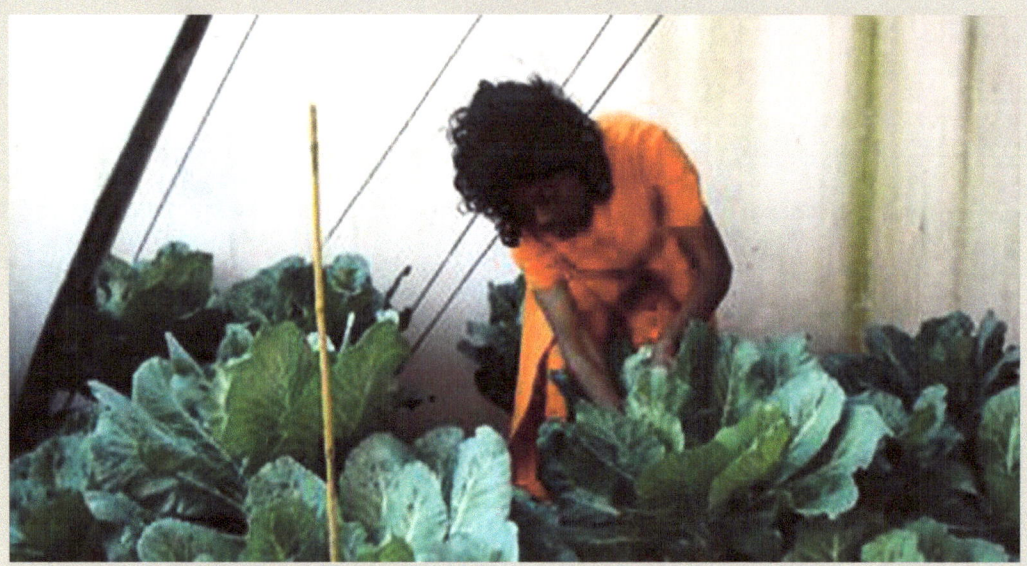

Her mother and grandmother both died of breast cancer at 47, and 36 years old, respectively. Her grandmother's sisters died of cancer at early ages. Diabetes runs in her family.

Annette Larkins is in perfect health and doesn't take aspirin. In fact, she doesn't take any medication at all, at least by the conventional modern definition. She is a fanatic of REAL medicine and lives by the quote, "Let food be thy medicine and medicine be thy food." — Hippocrates

Mrs. Larkins grows a plethora of fruit, vegetables, and herbs around and inside of her house. She collects rainwater and makes gallons of juice from what she grows. Wheatgrass is one of her specialties. She grows her own and drinks the juice regularly. Yet another anecdotal case of raw food and juicing providing overall health and endless youth.

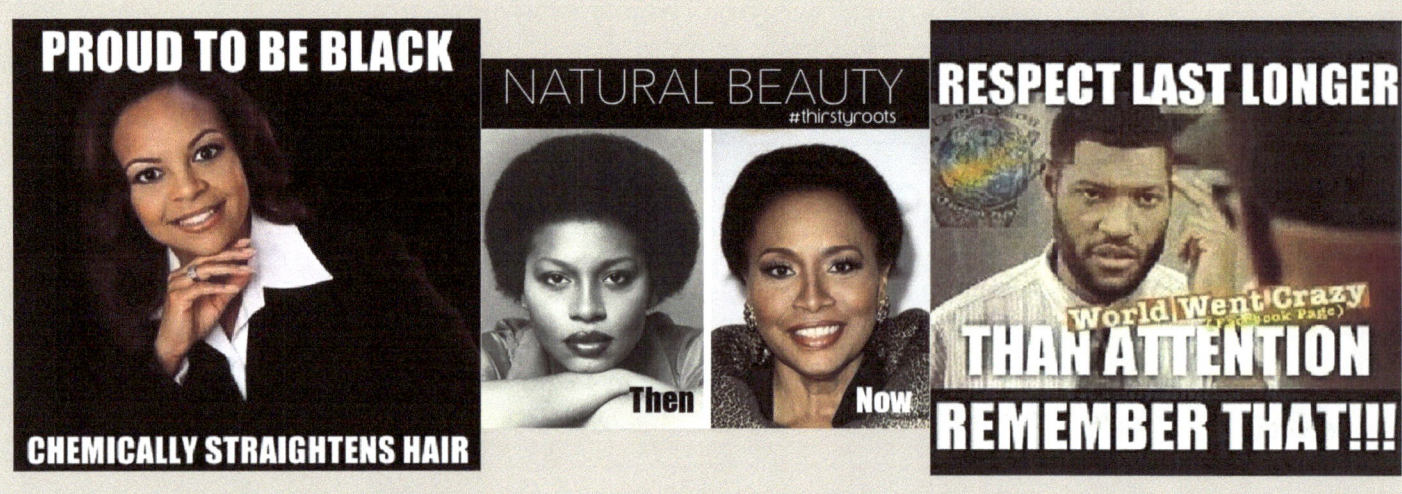

Black celebrities who should have their own workout videos

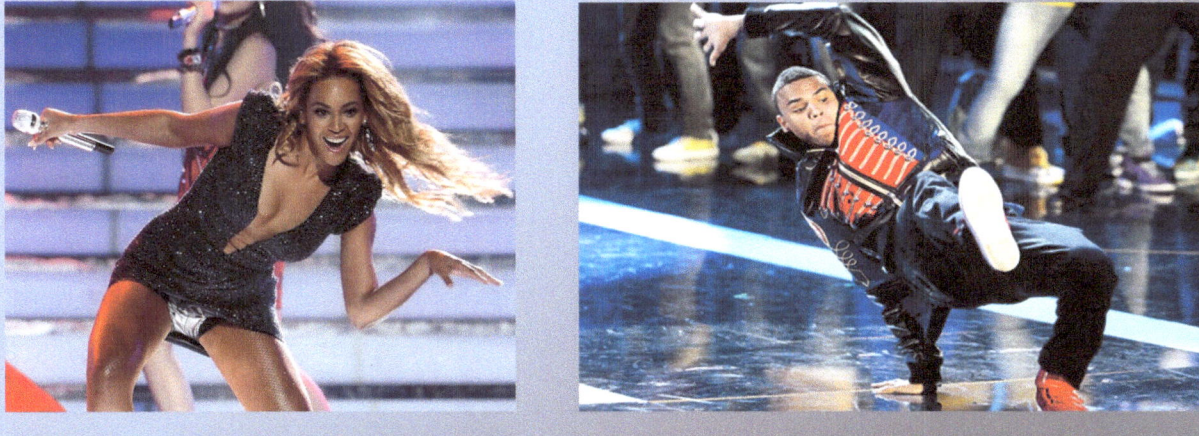

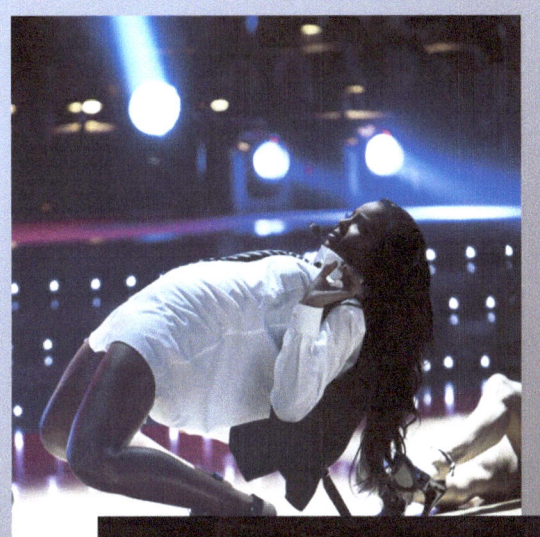

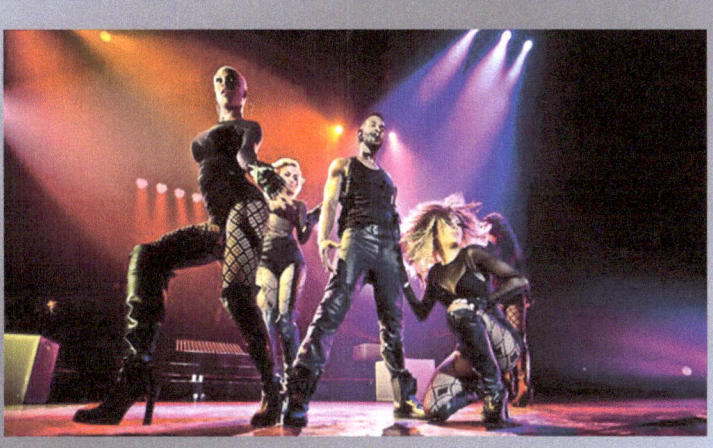

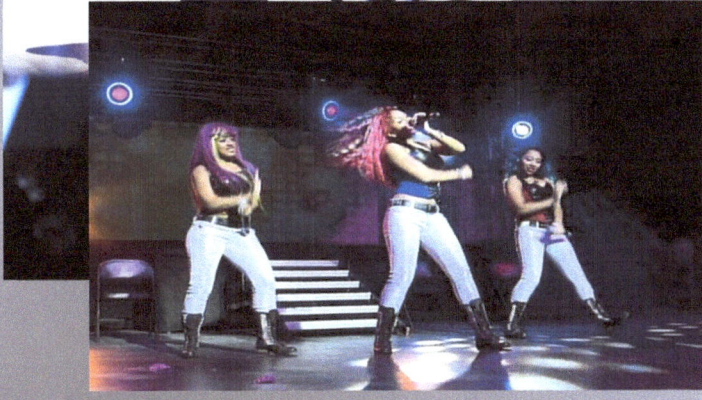

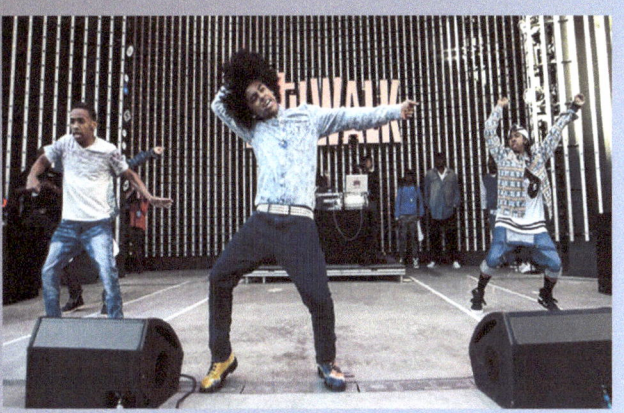

Beyonce   Chris Brown   Ciara   Usher   OMG   Mindless Behavior

We have all heard how Beyoncé runs on the treadmill in her heels and watched her shut the competition down with her dance moves. Now imagine Beyoncé moves on a workout video similar to "The Blackeye Pea Experience" or The Michael Jackson Experience" on the Wii.

Check out these celebs who not only have bangin' bodies but who also has the moves to help anyone dance off some pounds.

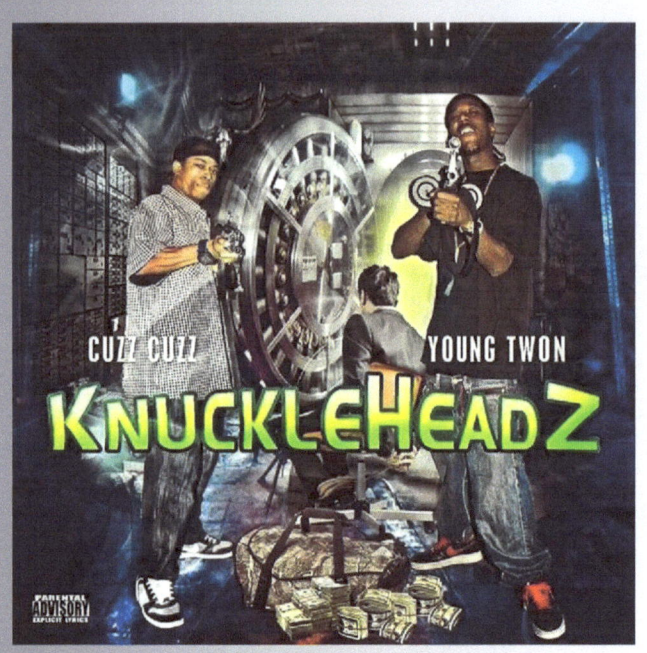

CUZZ CUZZ   YOUNG TWON
KNUCKLEHEADZ

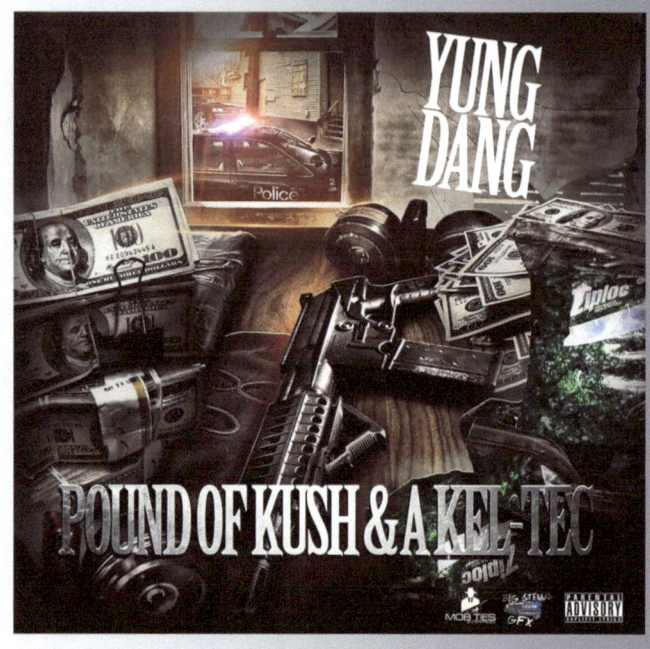

YUNG DANG
POUND OF KUSH & A KEL-TEC

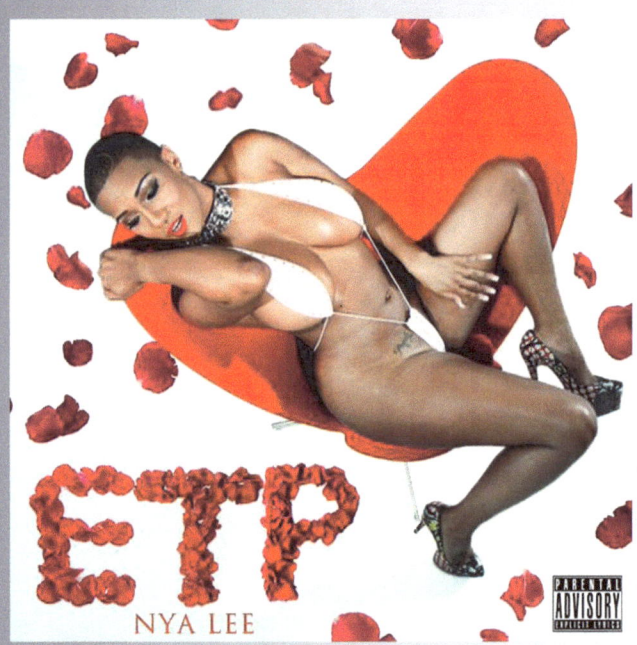

ETP
NYA LEE

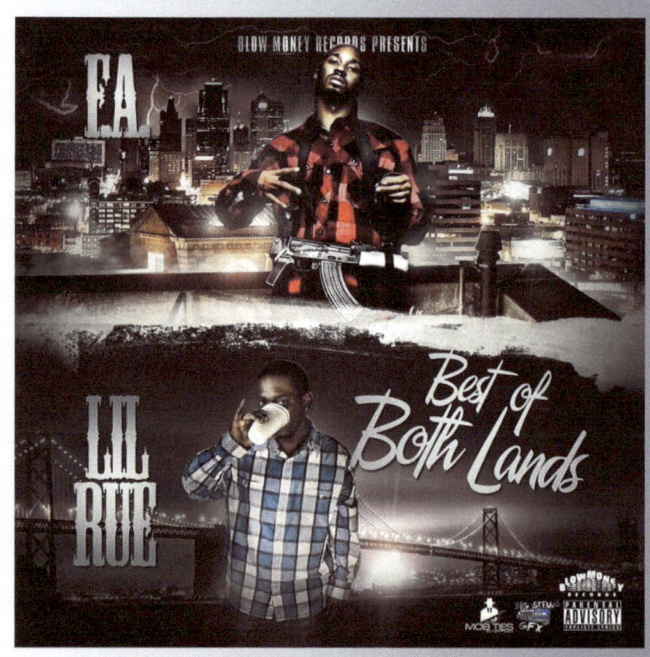

BLOW MONEY RECORDS PRESENTS
EA
LIL RUE
Best of Both Lands

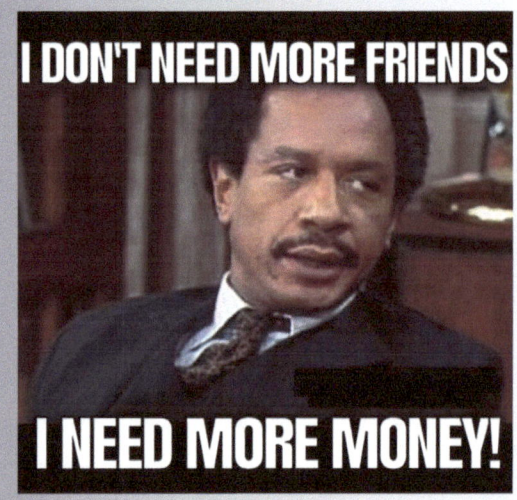

I DON'T NEED MORE FRIENDS

I NEED MORE MONEY!

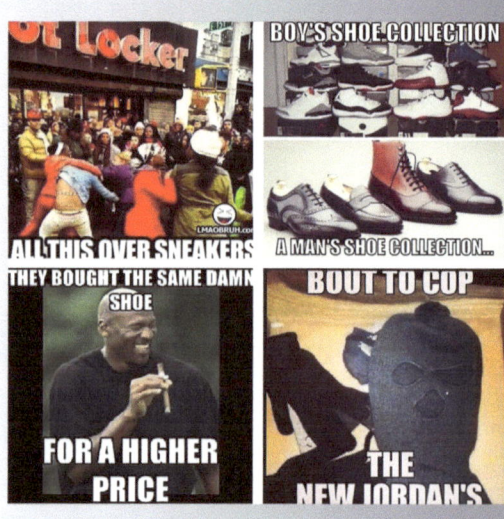

BOY'S SHOE COLLECTION

ALL THIS OVER SNEAKERS

A MAN'S SHOE COLLECTION...

THEY BOUGHT THE SAME DAMN SHOE
FOR A HIGHER PRICE

BOUT TO COP
THE NEW JORDAN'S

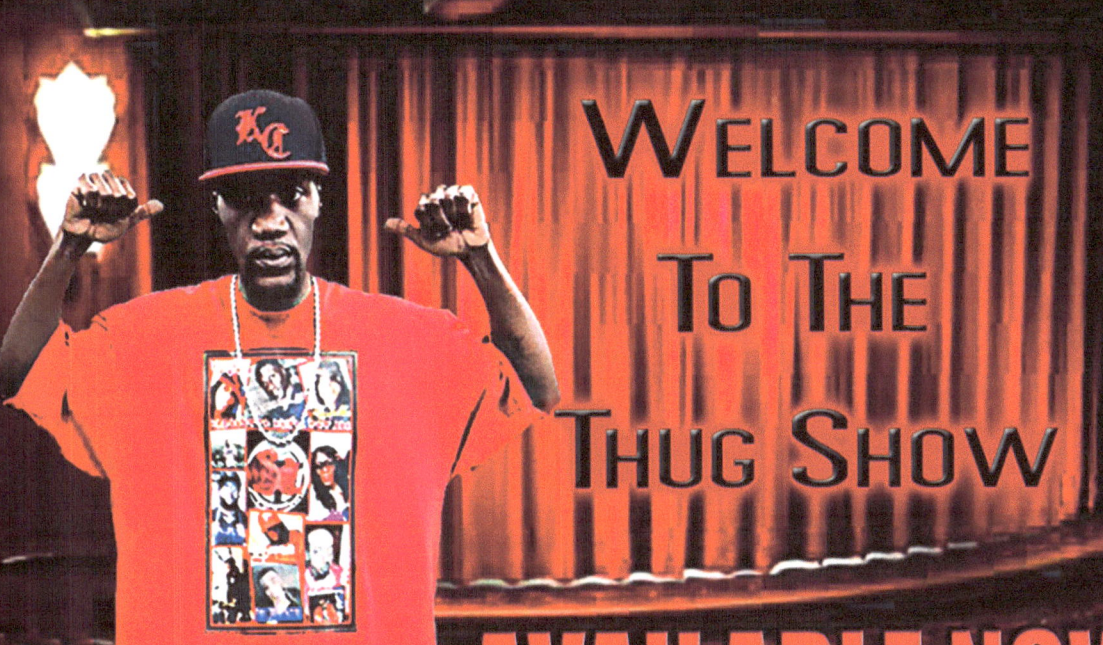
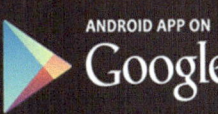

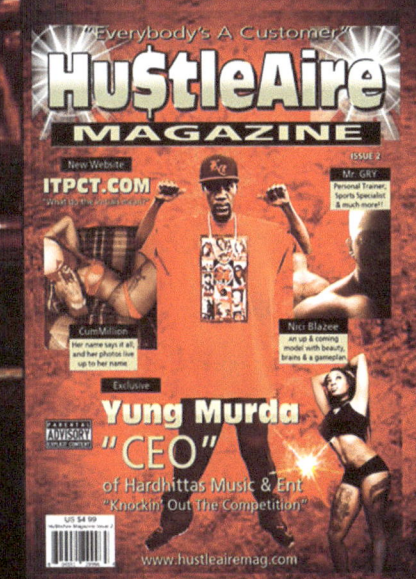
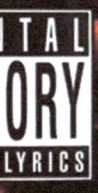

Sweet Capri

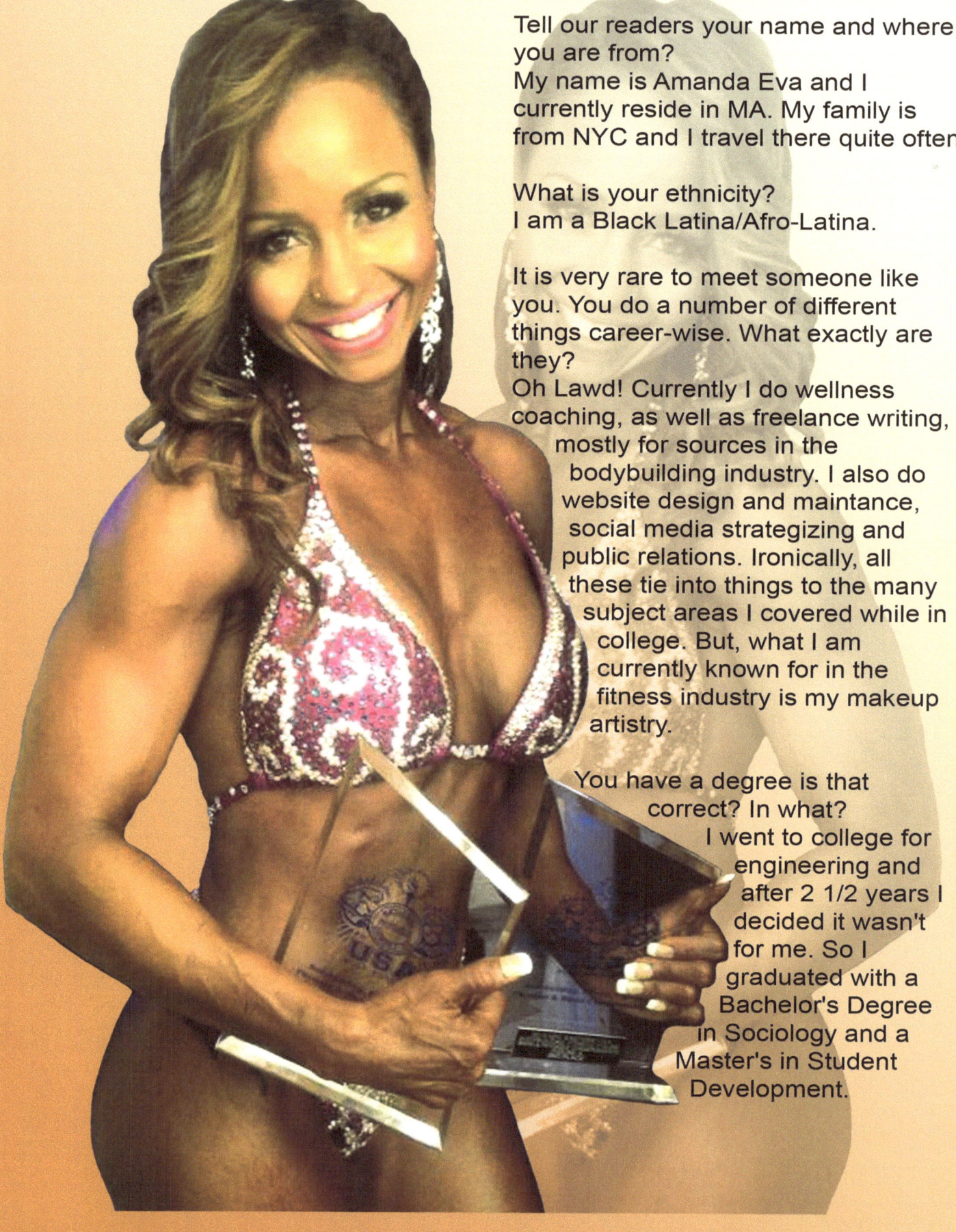

Tell our readers your name and where you are from?
My name is Amanda Eva and I currently reside in MA. My family is from NYC and I travel there quite often.

What is your ethnicity?
I am a Black Latina/Afro-Latina.

It is very rare to meet someone like you. You do a number of different things career-wise. What exactly are they?
Oh Lawd! Currently I do wellness coaching, as well as freelance writing, mostly for sources in the bodybuilding industry. I also do website design and maintance, social media strategizing and public relations. Ironically, all these tie into things to the many subject areas I covered while in college. But, what I am currently known for in the fitness industry is my makeup artistry.

You have a degree is that correct? In what?
I went to college for engineering and after 2 1/2 years I decided it wasn't for me. So I graduated with a Bachelor's Degree in Sociology and a Master's in Student Development.

In order to compete in physical fitness it takes a lot of hard work, training and discipline. What is and has been your motivation? I have tunnel vision. Once I set my goal to get on that stage, I just do it. I am constantly motivated by every woman around me who is able to keep up with the demands of their daily life and the rigor and discipline it takes to compete. I'm also my own motivation. While I know when to walk away, I don't quit easily.

You've coompeted in various bodybulding contest. How many have you done so far? I have done 11 figure competitions.

How often do you work out? When I'm getting ready to compete it's some serious business. I go to the gym up to 6 days per week, twice a day. The reason for doing this is because I break the cardio and training into 2 sessions, one cardio in the morning, and training and a little more cardio in the evenings. When I am not competing it varies on my goals for the upcoming season - for example, I am competing at the national level next year, so my training, even though it's not 6 days per week, it's about 5 days on average, with some cardio involved. I train with the same level of intensity year round.

Staying fit is a lifestyle. What are some things that whether you are training or not you won't eat? As far as unhealthy foods, I don't do fast foods restaurants often, Chipotle being an exception. I rarely eat red meat and if you ever bring a lobster near me we will have problems. I hate lobster. They look like giant sea roaches.

When I used to work out I would often do supersets. A push and a pull. What type of workout regimen do you do? I did that too many years ago! I train 1 to 2 body parts per training day. Right now I do bis and tris, legs, shoulders, back, and glute/hamstring day. I vary between going very heavy with low reps to moderate to light weights and high reps.

What are some of your favorite workout songs? "Money, Power, Respect" by the Lox, anything Beyonce, and Jay Z, old school hip hop - Biggie, Nas, etc.

How much can you bench? I don't bench press.

How much can you squat? Hmmm, I work out for definition not strength. But I think the highest might have been 200 something pounds.

What do you have in store for 2014? I'm looking forward to continuing my works as media strategist, build more client websites, and to continue my services as a makeup artist. I plan on getting back on the national stage since my last showing back in 2007 in hopes to earn pro status. Last but not least, I am having a birthday bash/official launch party around my birhday. More information will be posted on my FB page (Sweetcapri). You are invited!

How can you be contacted? I can most certainly be reached via my FB page (Sweetcapri) or via email at amanda@sweetcapri.com

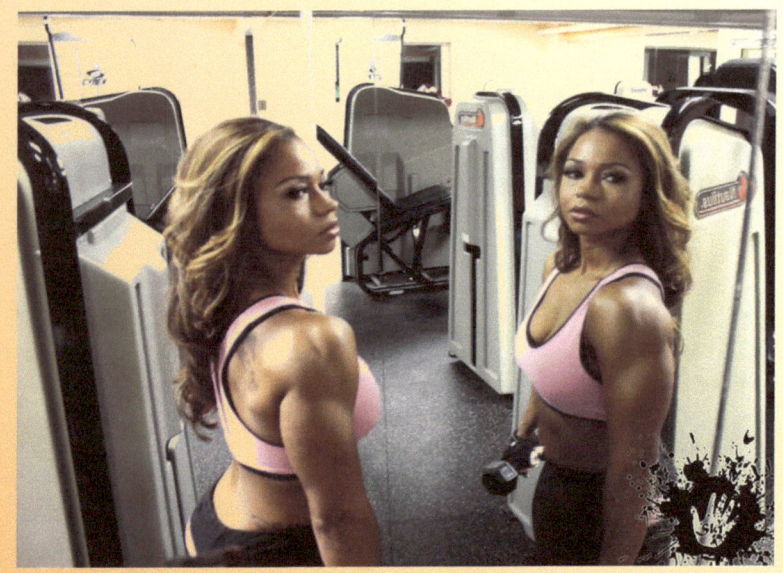
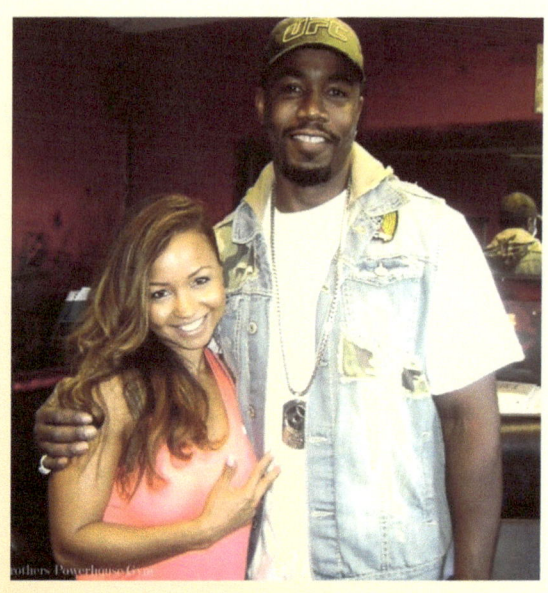
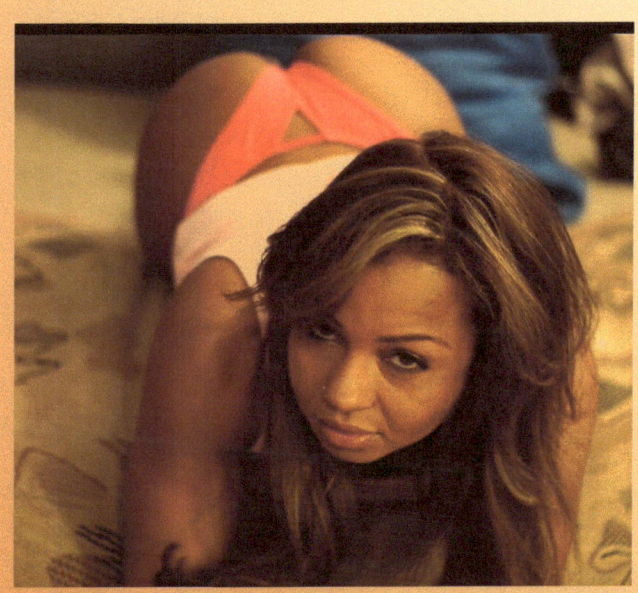
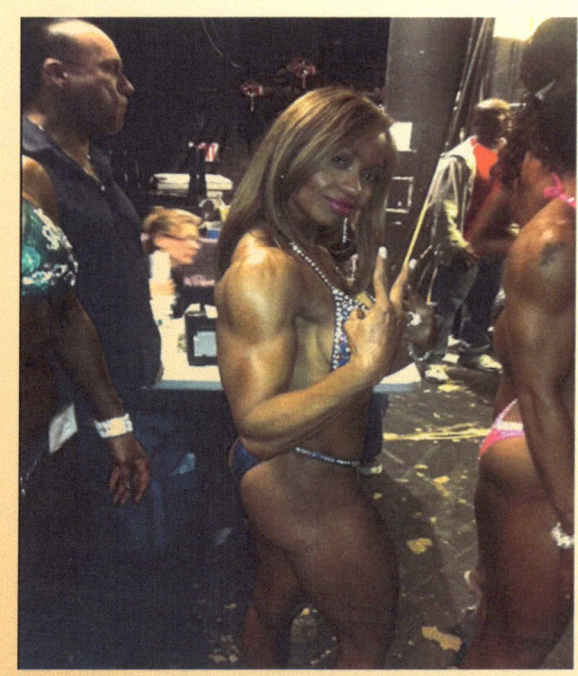
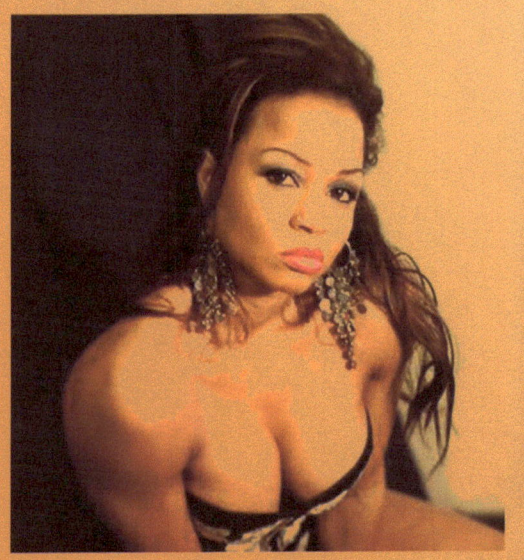
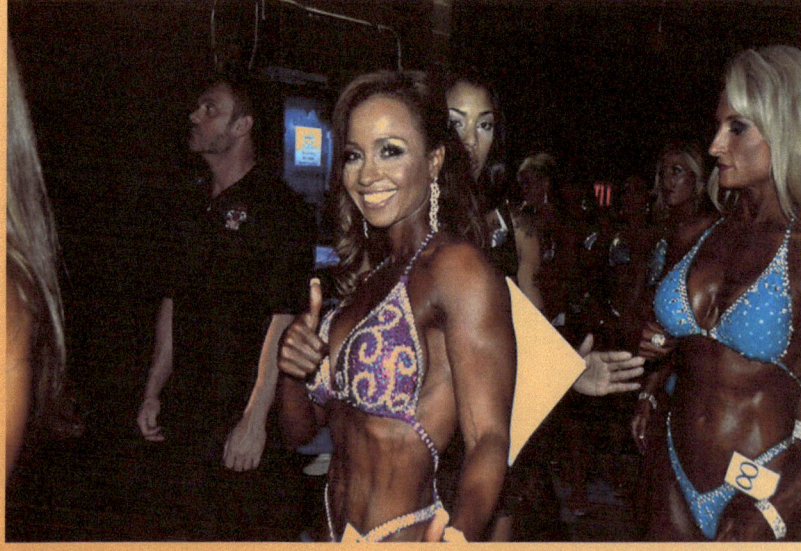

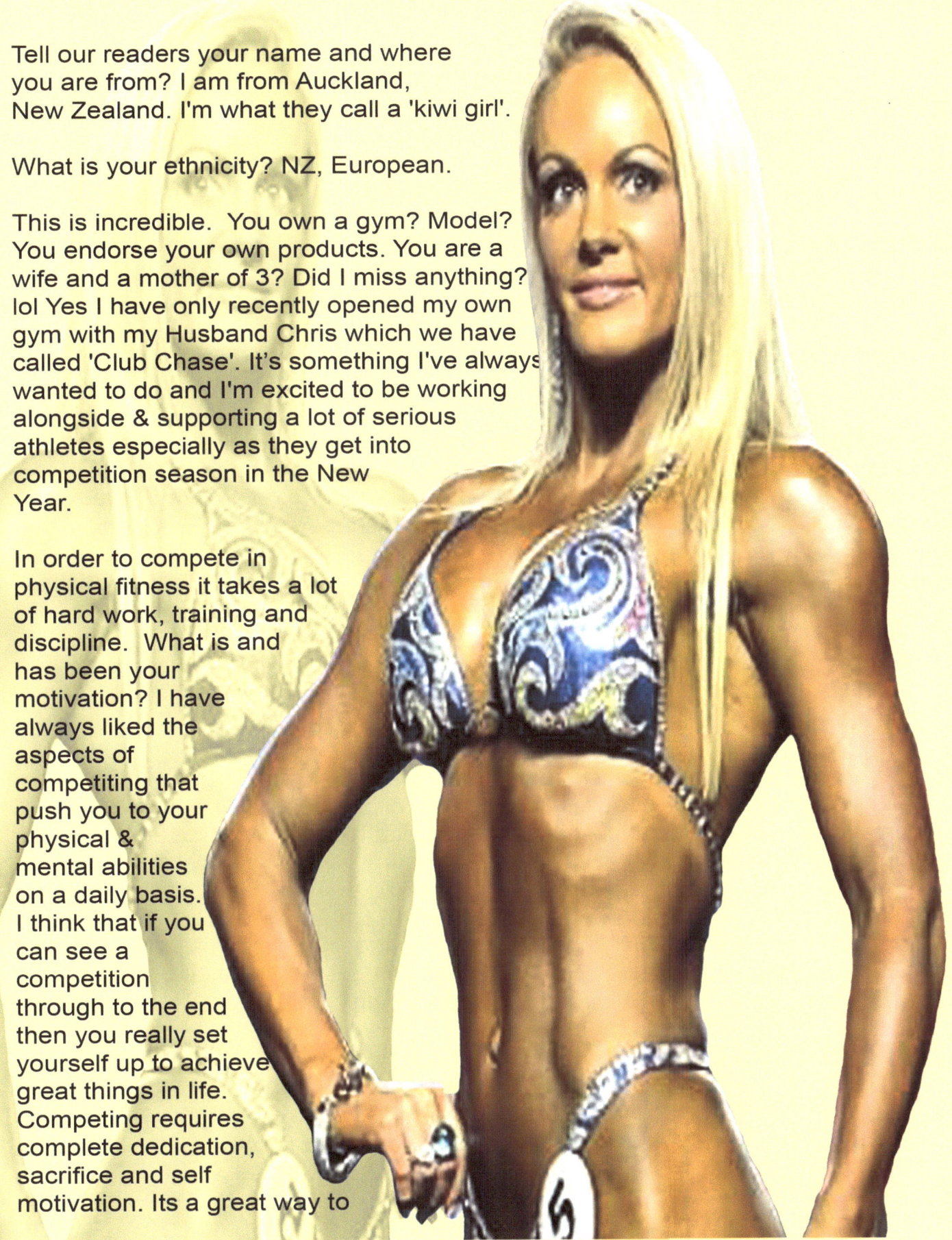

Raechelle Chase

Tell our readers your name and where you are from? I am from Auckland, New Zealand. I'm what they call a 'kiwi girl'.

What is your ethnicity? NZ, European.

This is incredible. You own a gym? Model? You endorse your own products. You are a wife and a mother of 3? Did I miss anything? lol Yes I have only recently opened my own gym with my Husband Chris which we have called 'Club Chase'. It's something I've always wanted to do and I'm excited to be working alongside & supporting a lot of serious athletes especially as they get into competition season in the New Year.

In order to compete in physical fitness it takes a lot of hard work, training and discipline. What is and has been your motivation? I have always liked the aspects of competiting that push you to your physical & mental abilities on a daily basis. I think that if you can see a competition through to the end then you really set yourself up to achieve great things in life. Competing requires complete dedication, sacrifice and self motivation. Its a great way to

You've competed in various bodybulding contest. How many have you done so far? During my Professional Carer, I have competed in 8 Professional International competitions including being the 1st NZ Figure Athlete to compete in the Figure Olympia in 2011 which is a huge achievement that I am very proud of.

How often do you work out?
Training intensity changes depending on where I am at in terms of which competitions I am aiming for. Each contest prep is carefully planned out to ensure I am stage ready by the required date. In the off season, I maintain my figure & body fat levels by training 5-6 days per week. I don't do much cardio when I am not prepping for a show. Cardio is easily the least favorite part of getting in shape for me but unfortunately the most important when leaning down for a contest. I believe that with good nutrition and regular weight training, daily cardio is NOT essential in maintaining a nice toned body that you can keep in shape all year round. I generally aim to do cardio 3 times a week for 45 mins at a time.

Staying fit is a lifestyle. What are some things that whether you are training or not you won't eat? Because being fit & healthy should be something you strive to make your lifestyle, I don't deprive myself of any particular kinds of food. The old saying everything in moderation though it sounds cliche is definitely the key to enjoying life without going overboard with binge eating marathons. I don't believe that its ever 'too late' to get in shape or start on the road to being healthy, but it's definitely easier to stay in shape than it is to get in shape. Taking the time to prepare healthy meals for yourself and your family, and keeping active should be a priority. If you have health you have hope. If you have hope you have everything.

What are some of your favorite workout songs?
In terms of music, I'm not too fussy, as long as it's loud and energetic I am happy. I love training. It doesn't take a lot to motivate me once I'm in the gym. Often the hardest part of training is just getting to the gym!

How much can you bench? I don't bench press :) My heaviest squat is 100kgs, low & slow. Squats are an essential exercise to building muscle on your legs. It's important to get the basics right with your squatting technique before loading the machine up with super heavy weights to avoid injury.

What do you have in store for 2014? To be honest, I'm not sure yet, I am by nature a very impulsive person, I'm always looking for fun, adventerous new opportunities to keep life interesting. At the same time I'm a huge believer in setting goals. learning from each experience and growing spiritually as I go.

How can you be contacted? FACE BOOK: Raechelle Chase
WEBSITE: www.raechellechase.com
INSTAGRAM: http://instagram.com/raechellechase
YOU TUBE: http://www.youtube.com/user/raechellechase
TWITTER: https://twitter.com/RaechelleChase

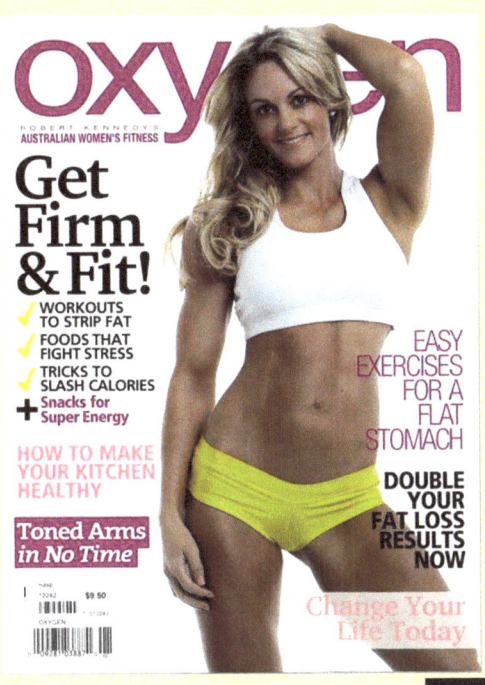

OXY en

ROBERT KENNEDY'S
AUSTRALIAN WOMEN'S FITNESS

Get Firm & Fit!

- ✓ WORKOUTS TO STRIP FAT
- ✓ FOODS THAT FIGHT STRESS
- ✓ TRICKS TO SLASH CALORIES
- ✚ Snacks for Super Energy

HOW TO MAKE YOUR KITCHEN HEALTHY

Toned Arms in No Time

$9.50

OXYGEN

EASY EXERCISES FOR A FLAT STOMACH

DOUBLE YOUR FAT LOSS RESULTS NOW

Change Your Life Today

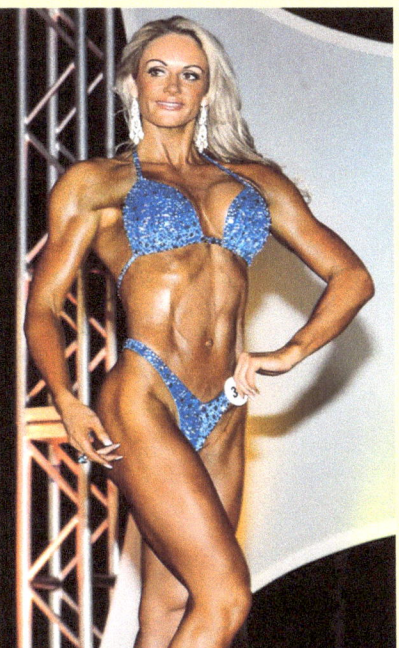

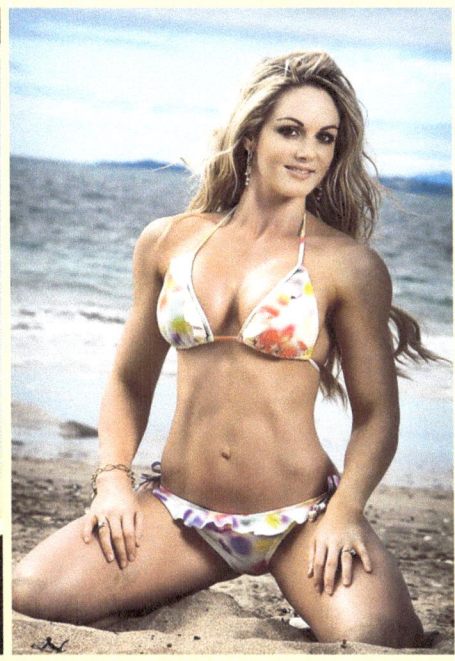

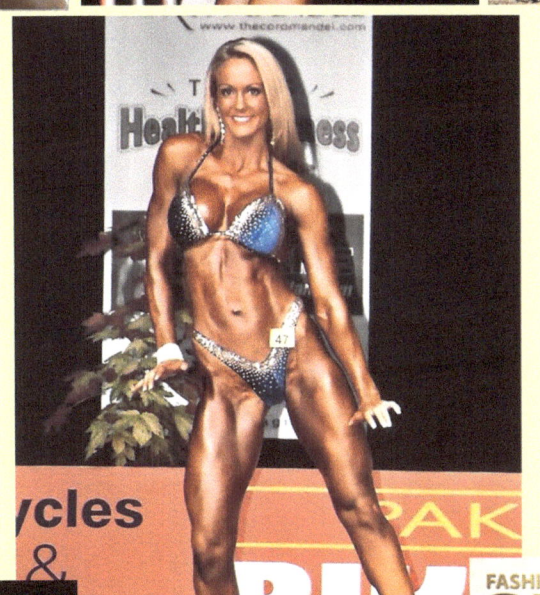

www.thecoromandel.com

Health ness

cycles & ers

PAK

BIKE

47

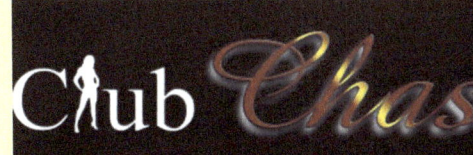

Club Chase

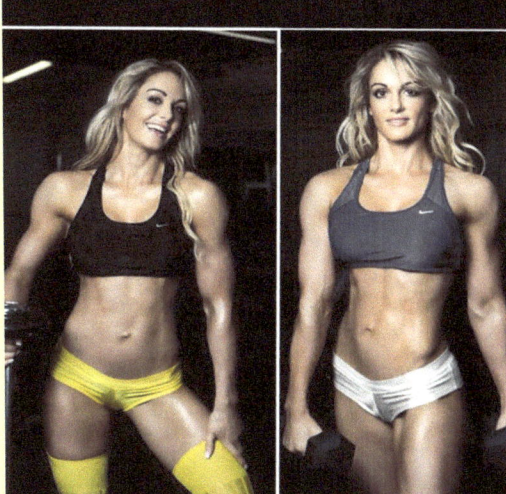

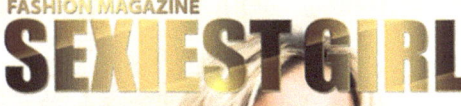

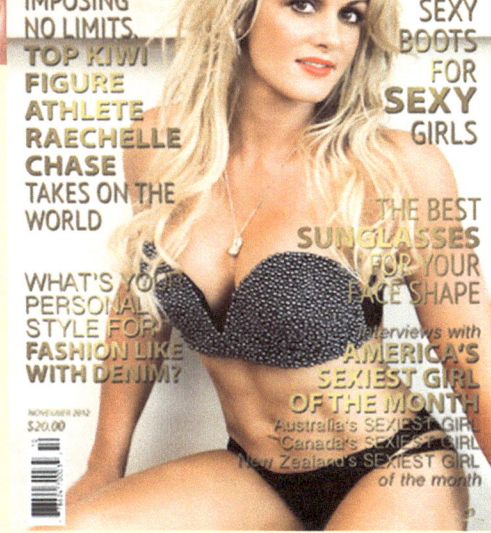

FASHION MAGAZINE

SEXIEST GIRL

IMPOSING NO LIMITS, **TOP KIWI FIGURE ATHLETE RAECHELLE CHASE** TAKES ON THE WORLD

WHAT'S YOUR PERSONAL STYLE FOR FASHION LIKE WITH DENIM?

SEXY BOOTS FOR SEXY GIRLS

THE BEST SUNGLASSES FOR YOUR FACE SHAPE

Interviews with **AMERICA'S SEXIEST GIRL OF THE MONTH** Australia's SEXIEST GIRL Canada's SEXIEST GIRL New Zealand's SEXIEST GIRL of the month

NOVEMBER 2012

$20.00

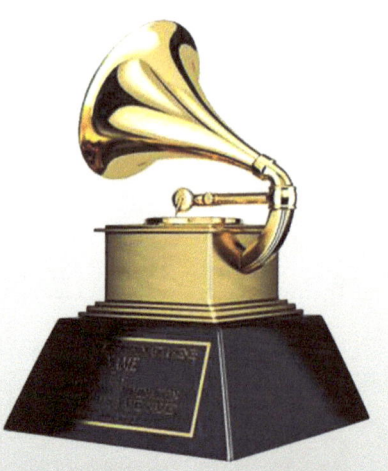

2014 Grammy Awards

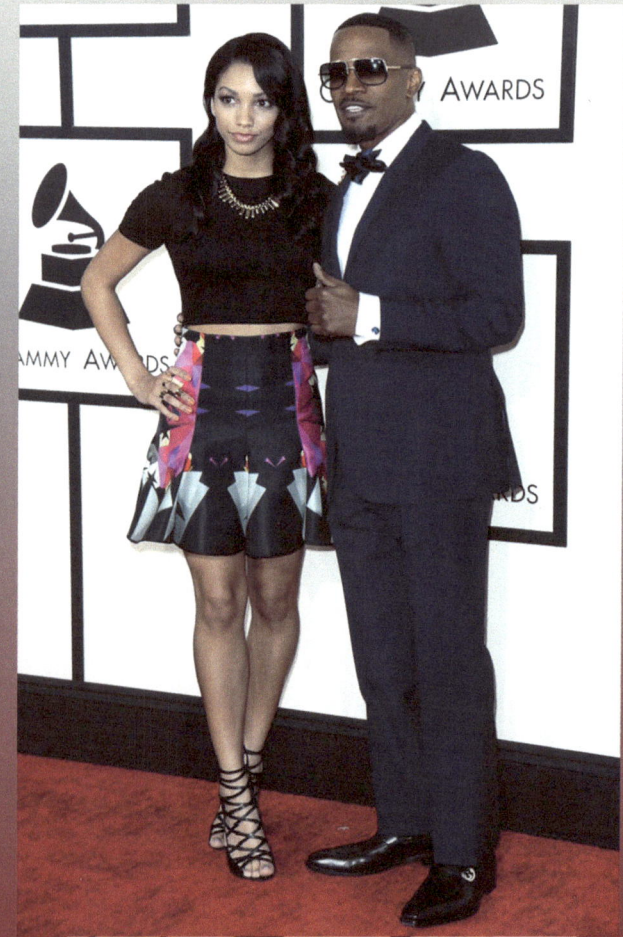

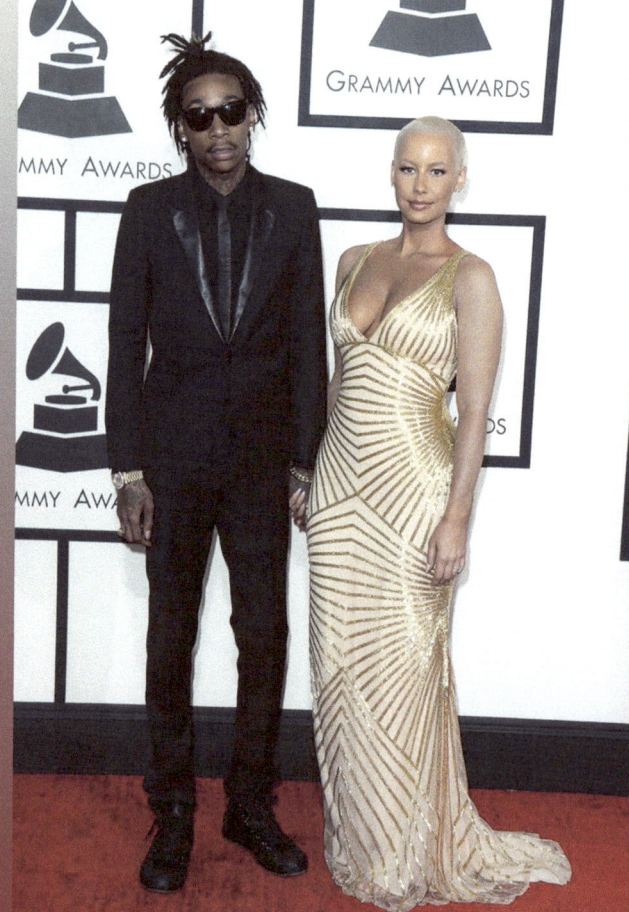

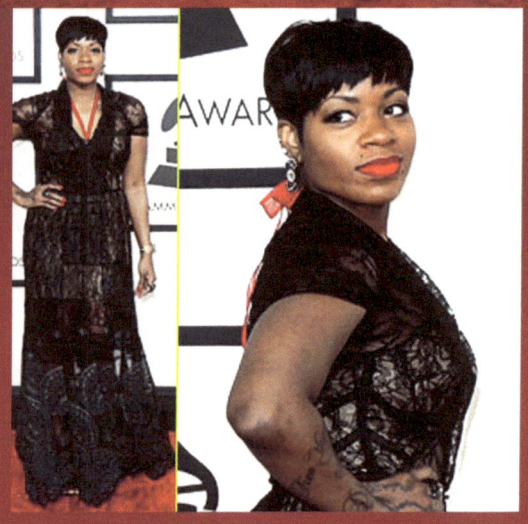

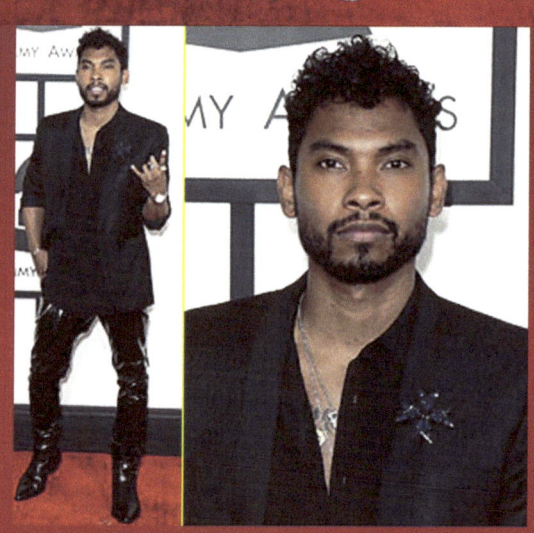

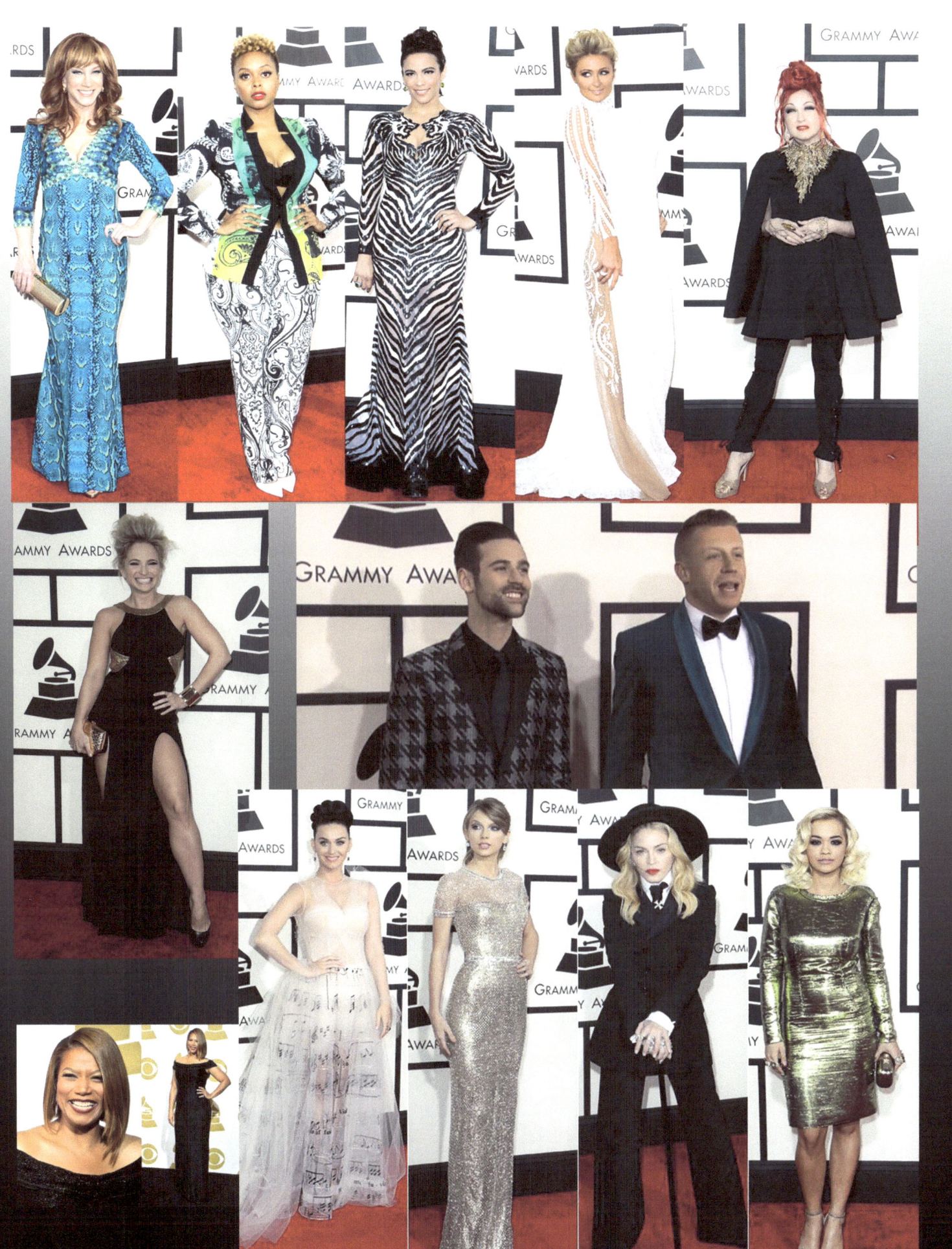

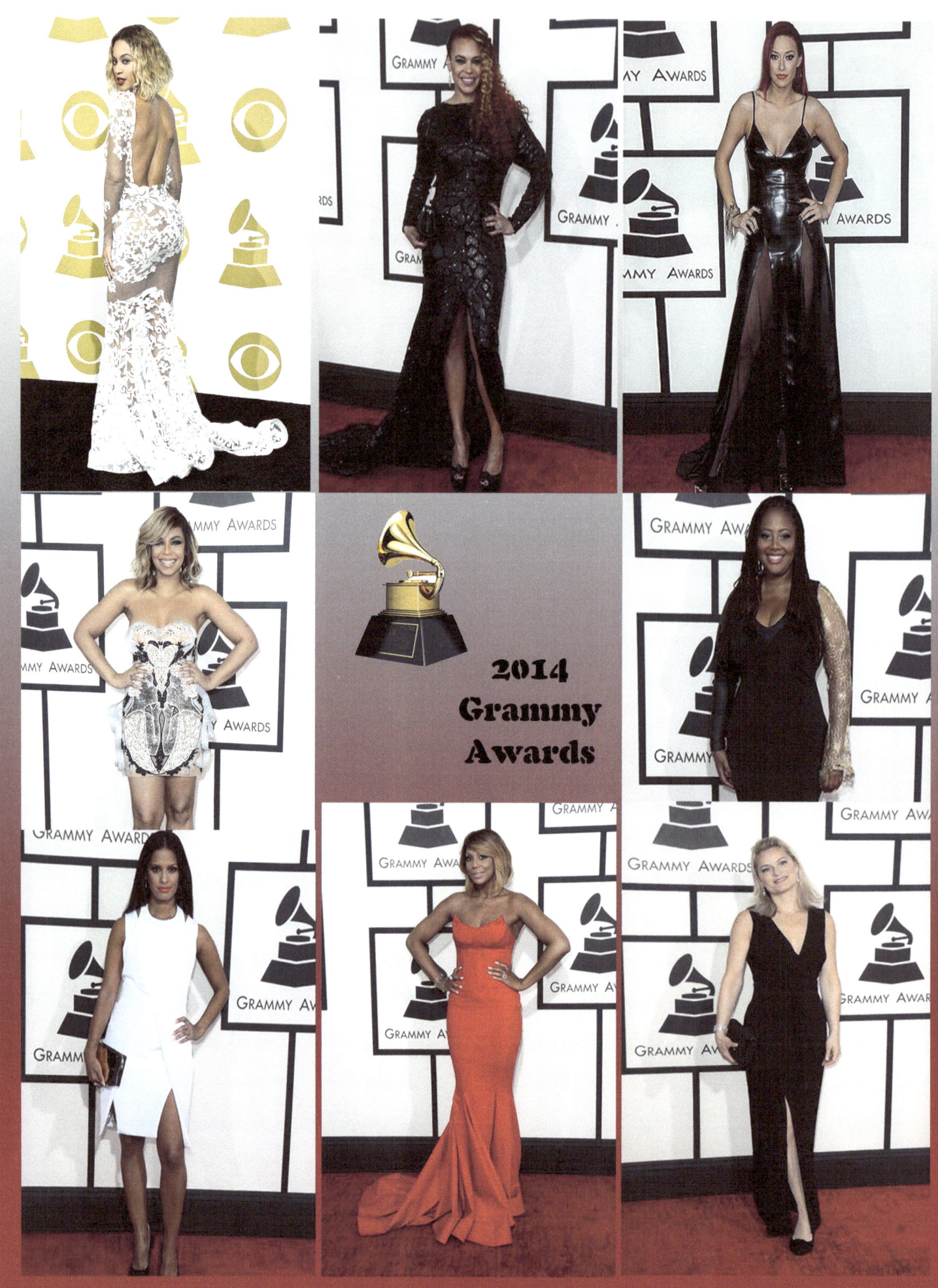

2014
Grammy
Awards

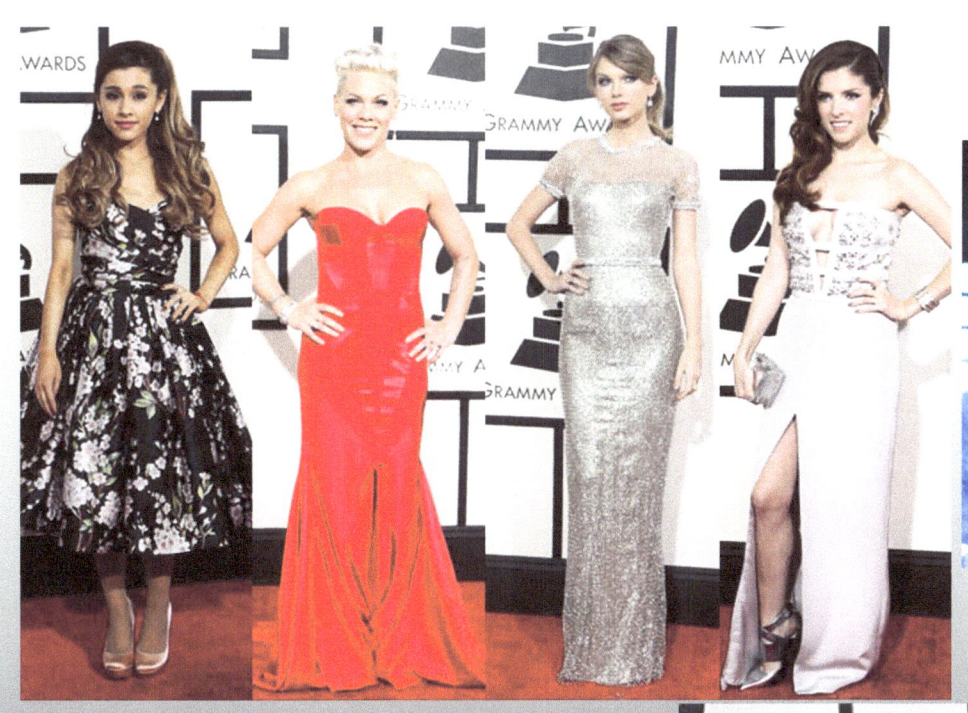

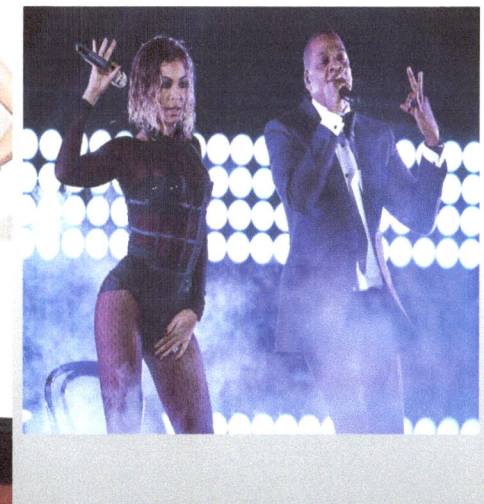

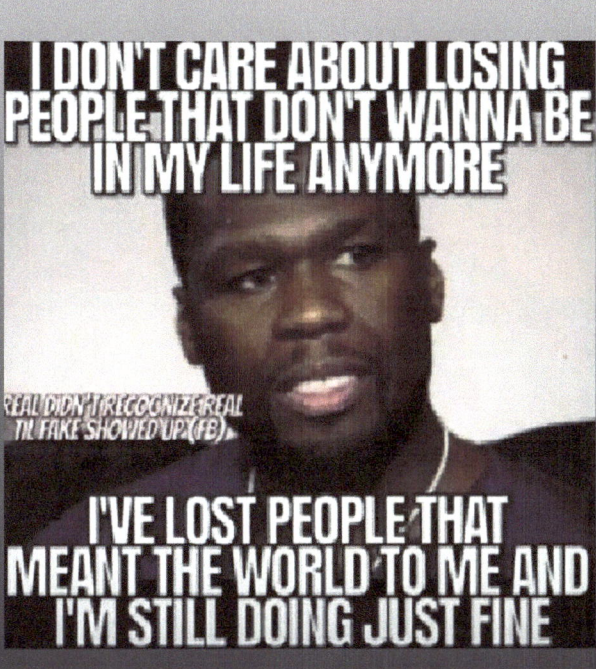

I DON'T CARE ABOUT LOSING PEOPLE THAT DON'T WANNA BE IN MY LIFE ANYMORE

REAL DIDN'T RECOGNIZE REAL TIL FAKE SHOWED UP (FB)

I'VE LOST PEOPLE THAT MEANT THE WORLD TO ME AND I'M STILL DOING JUST FINE

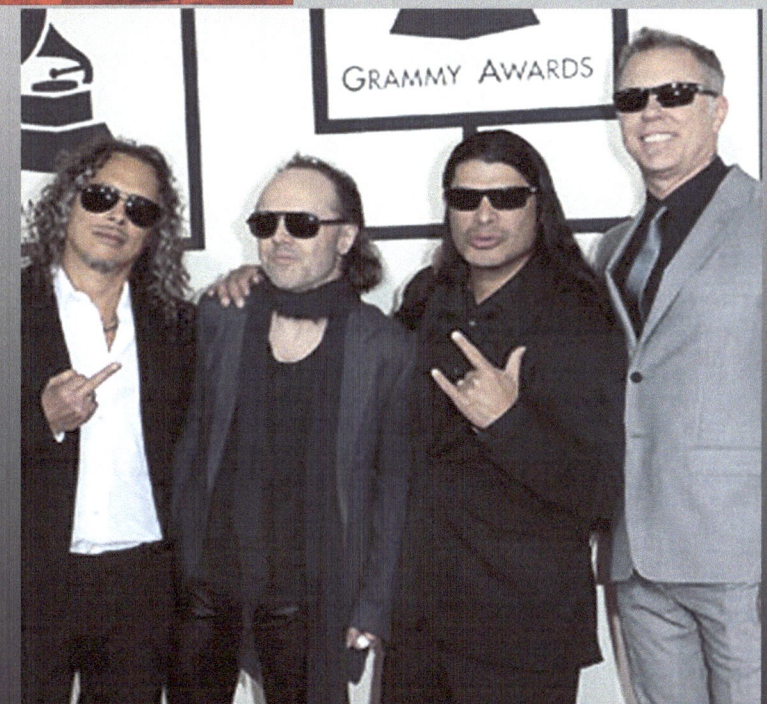

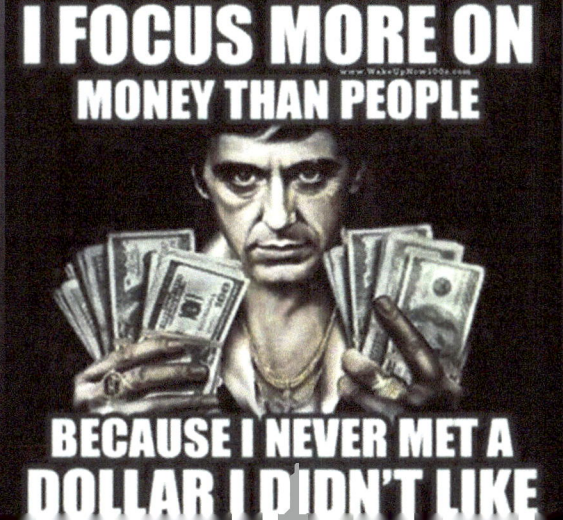

I FOCUS MORE ON MONEY THAN PEOPLE

www.WakeUpNow100x.com

BECAUSE I NEVER MET A DOLLAR I DIDN'T LIKE

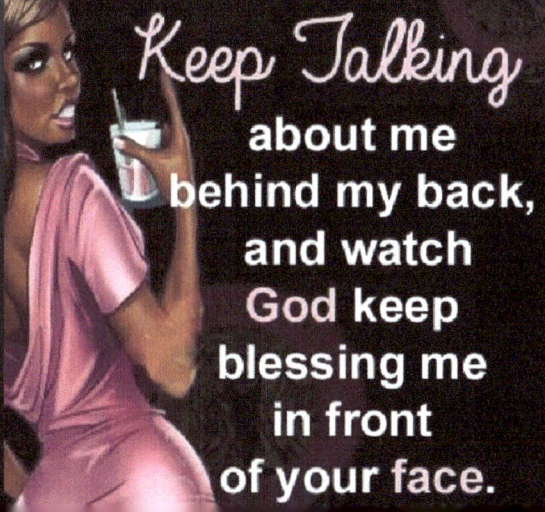

Keep Talking about me behind my back, and watch God keep blessing me in front of your face.

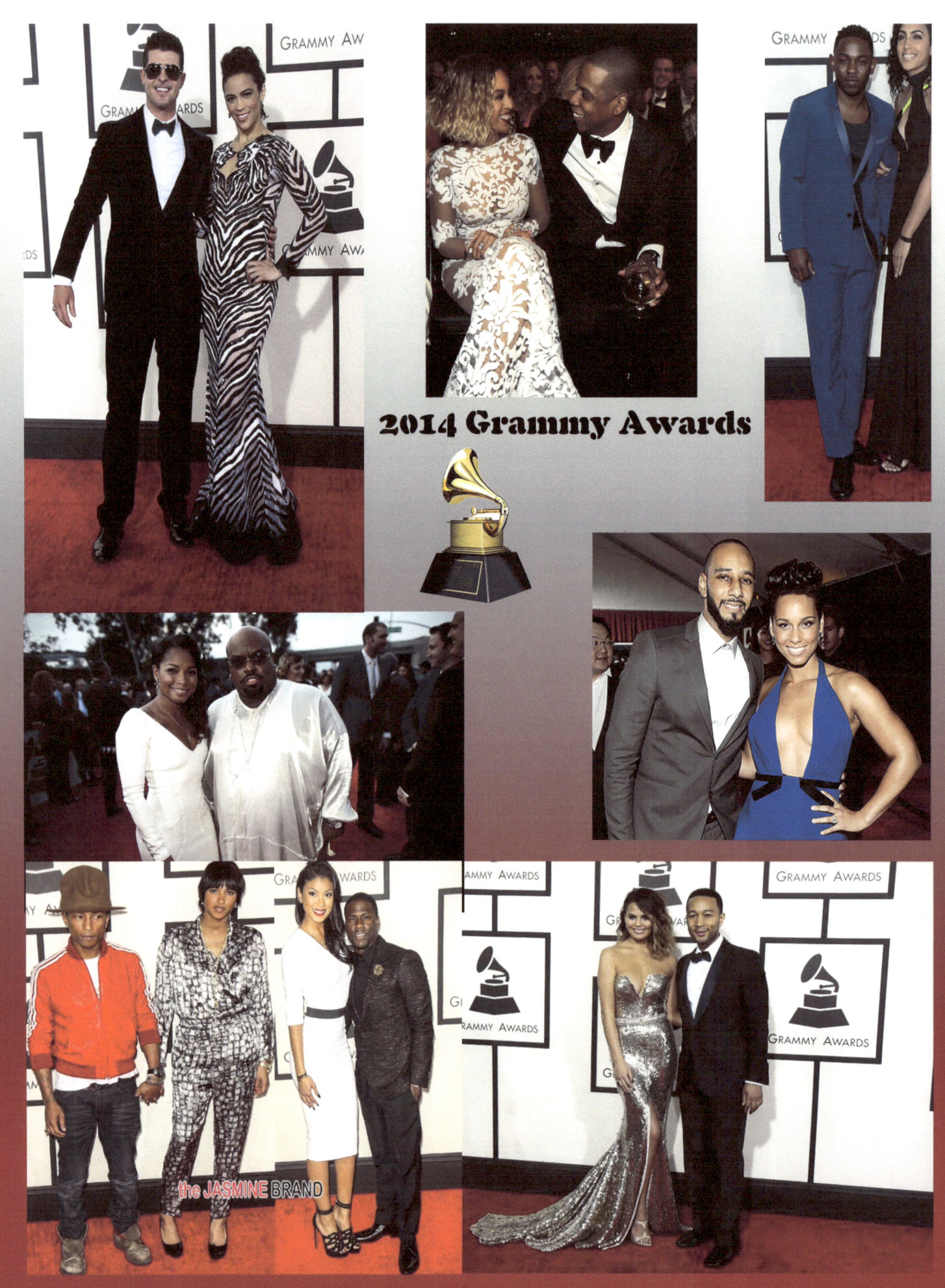

2014 Grammy Awards

Your Hip-Hop Workout Playlist

Your Hip-Hop Workout Playlist

Motivation is the key to keeping you primed to keep pushing heavy weight in the gym. And what better motivator is there than music? We asked the experts—our dedicated Muscle & Fitness fans—what workout songs makes their heart rate rise and gets them pumped to hit new PRs, and you answered. If you prefer hip-hop beats to get your muscles primed for a full-on assault, here are 25 rap songs for your workout playlist.

This also appears in Muscle and Fitness

1. Lapdance – N.E.R.D.
2. Soldier – Eminem
3. Throw It Up – Lil Jon
4. Ambitionz az a Ridah – Tupac
5. N***as in Paris – Jay-Z and Kanye West
6. Bring the Pain – Method Man
7. We Right Here – DMX
8. Work Hard Play Hard – Wiz Khalifa
9. Good Feeling – Flo Rida
10. Hit 'Em Up – Tupac
11. Go Get It – T.I.
12. F**kin' Problems - A$AP Rocky
13. Hero – Nas
14. Push It – Rick Ross
15. Stronger – Kanye West
16. Jump Around – House of Pain
17. Not Afraid – Eminem
18. Pushin' Weight – Ice Cube
19. Hold Strong – Rob Bailey & the Hustle Standard
20. We Made It – Busta Rhymes Feat. Linkin Park
21. Rollin' – Limp Bizkit Feat. DMX
22. Rock Superstar – Cypress Hill
23. Hold Me Back – Rick Ross
24. The Uppercut – Tupac
25. Ali Bomaye – The Game

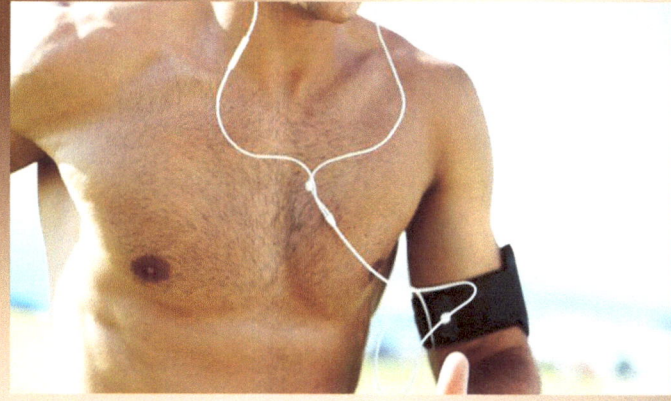

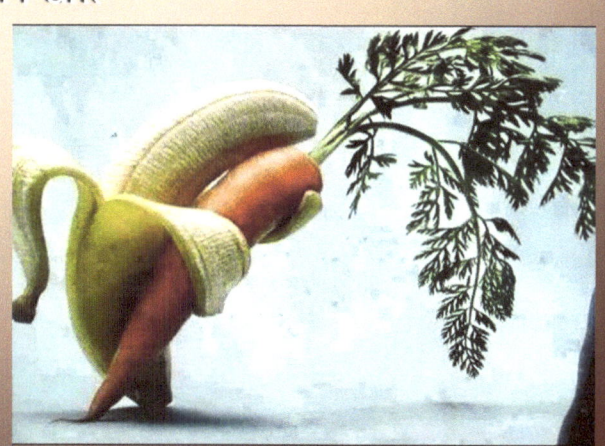

AL-BUM / MIXTAPE REVIEW

Riv Locc-Killer Instinct

Date Released: Jan 17, 2014

Genre: Hip-Hop/R&B, Style: Rap

Label: Reality Records / CD Baby

Total Tracks: 19   Total Length: 65:43

Tracklisting...
1. Intro
2. Natraul Born Mobsta
3. Don't Belive
(feat. Luni Coleone & Boy Geneyus)
4. I'm a Monsta (feat. Rico)
5. Gladiator (feat. Mr.4000 & Tanquara Locc)
6. Keep It Gangsta (feat. Reece Locc & Mr. Shaky)
7. Interlude (feat. Mac Blast)
8. Fucking Up My Weekend
(feat. Mississippi & Pacman Reese)
9. Murder in My Jean (feat. Young Ant Da Maniac & Mon Eg)
10. Same O Niggaz (feat. Steve Yancey, Blocc Monsta & Raymacc)
11. She Don't Like Me (feat. Sic Wit It & Jdiggs)
12. Slice of the Devils Pie
13. Get Dirty (feat. Stylion & Bull Locc)
14. Killer Instinct (feat. Zoo)
15. Not Like Me (feat. Rico)
16. PDA Thizzkidd Interlude
17. On My Mamma (feat. Ron Ron, Ric Raw & Philthy Fats)
18. One
19. Hypathetically Speaking

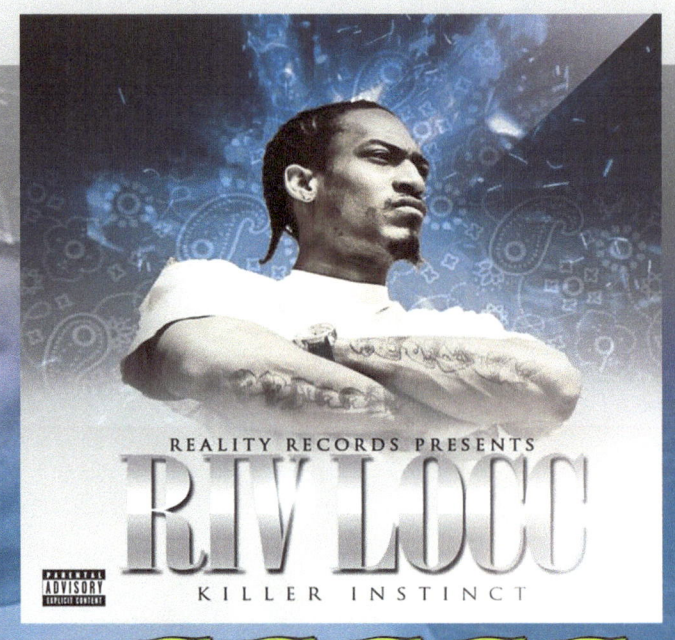

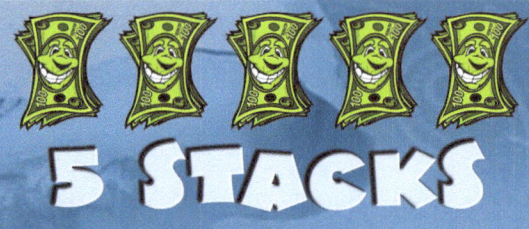

5 STACKS

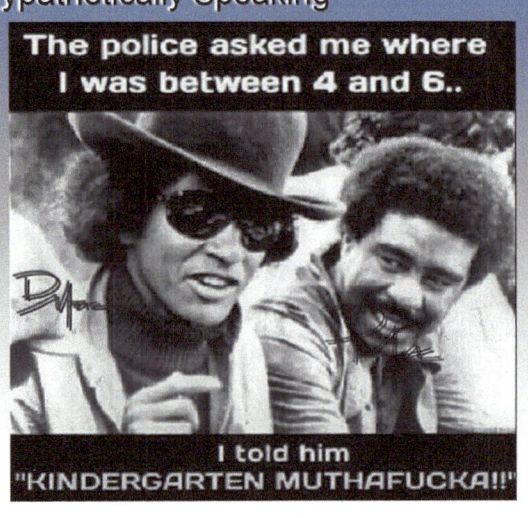

The police asked me where I was between 4 and 6..

I told him
"KINDERGARTEN MUTHAFUCKA!!"

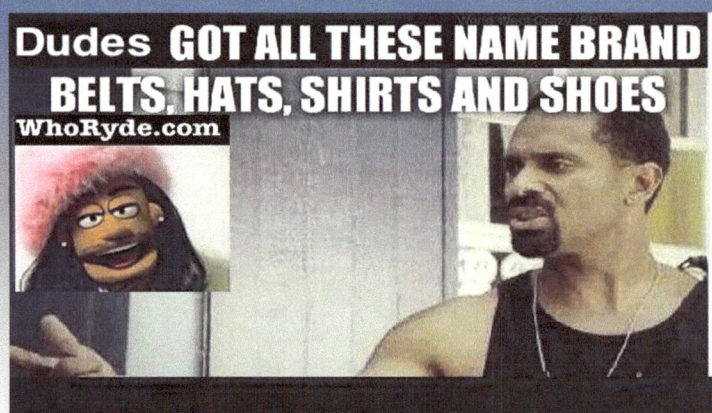

Dudes **GOT ALL THESE NAME BRAND BELTS, HATS, SHIRTS AND SHOES**

WhoRyde.com

But got a public defender as their lawyer!

"Everybody's A Customer"

Hu$tleAire
MAGAZINE

Hu$tleaire Magazine is looking for writers, sales reps, sponsors, ad contributors, models, artist and entrepreneurs.

IF YOU ARE INTERESTED PLEASE CONTACT US:

www.hustleairemag.com

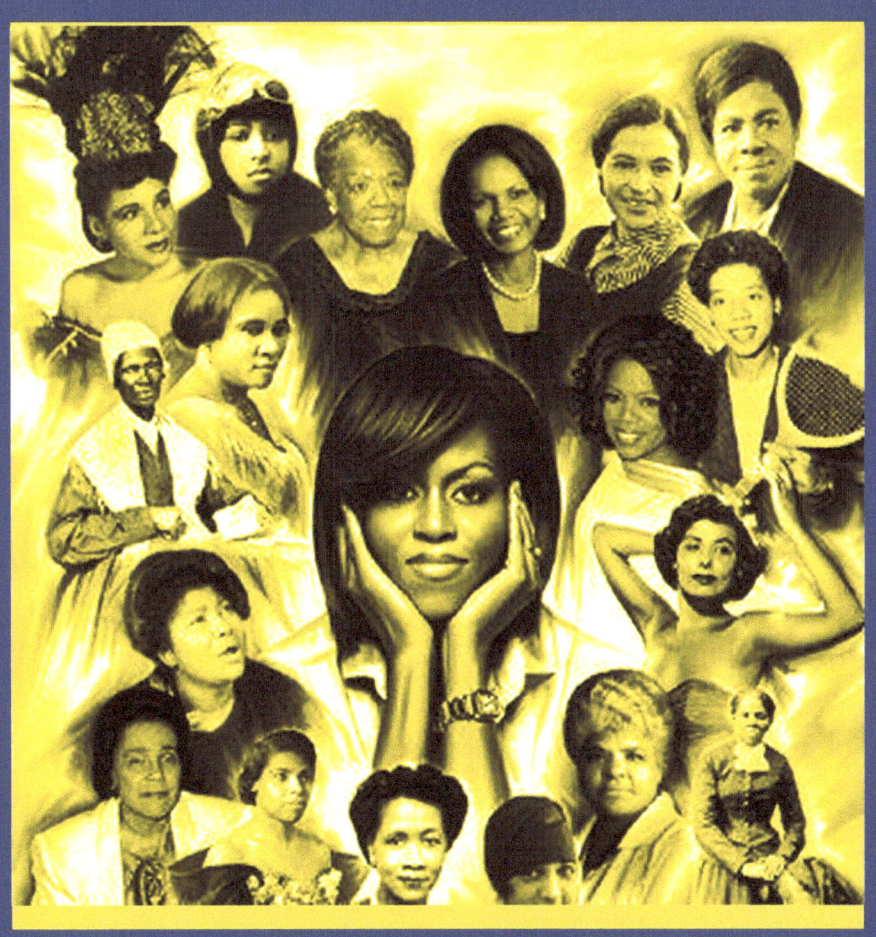

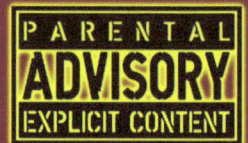
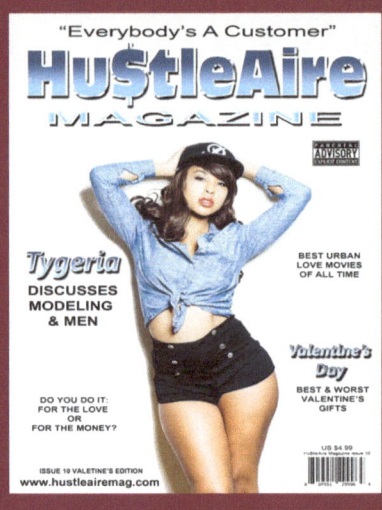
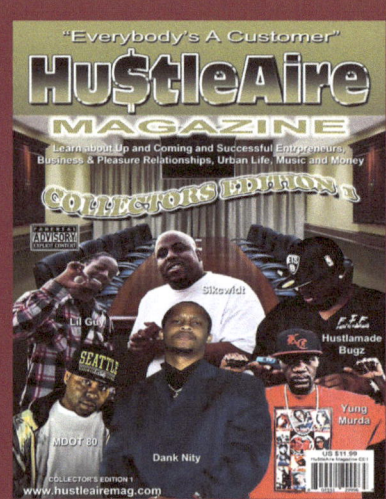
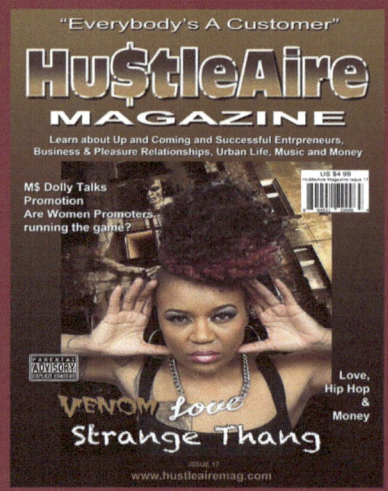
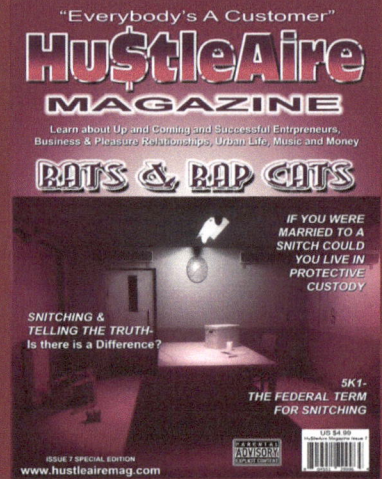
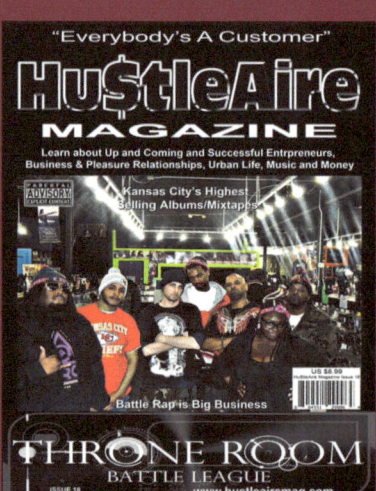
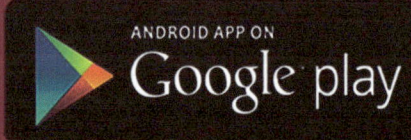